The Fast Diet
Magic Book

First Edition

Cover Design by Michael Warren

The author and publisher of this material make no medical claims for its use. This material is not intended to treat, diagnose nor cure any illness. If you need medical attention, please consult your doctor.

The Fast Diet Magic Book

The Cheat's Guide to Easy Weight Loss with Intermittent Fasting

Caitlin Collins

For the hungry ones

CONTENTS

1 WHY ALL THE HYPE ABOUT FAST DIETING?

Like most people who watched Michael Mosley's BBC TV show, *Eat, Fast and Live Longer*, I was immediately excited and even inspired by the idea of 'dieting' for only two days per week, eating normally for those other five, and still losing a ton of weight. I watched as Michael lost almost a stone (14lbs) in eight weeks. I saw how easy he found it. I noted how he had to go down to fasting just one day out of seven, in order not to get too thin.

And so, I began. My husband and I, both equally inspired, began fasting just two days a week – having only 500 calories on this day (he had 600) –

and waited for results. For my husband, it was an instant success. He lost from the first fast, and a steady 2-3lbs a week simply fell off him.

But for me, things weren't quite so straightforward. One month in to the plan and I hadn't lost a single pound and I hadn't cheated *once!* In these early days, I was reliant on pre-packaged Weight Watcher meals so there was no danger of my having inadvertently overeaten. After two months, I was ready to give up. This 5:2 fast diet just didn't work for me. Still despondent about my weight, which was two stone (28lbs) heavier than I would have liked, I went back to the old diets for a quick fix of fast weight loss – I did a few weeks of Atkins low-carb diet. I did a juice fast (I have never known hunger like those ten days!) I tried Tim Ferris's *Four Hour Body* Diet. And I lost some weight with all of them – about ten pounds overall. But life began to get in the way of consistent dieting, and in January of this year, after a particularly decadent Christmas, I jumped on the scales and discovered I was heavier than I had ever been at 11st 6lbs. Unbelievably, this was heavier than the 11st 2lbs I had weighed when 9 months pregnant.

I had no motivation to start a new faddy diet this time. I was so fed up with cutting out *this*, or eating tiny portions of *that*. I tried, and tried, and *tried* to cut down my carbohydrate intake. I had done my best to avoid wheat and sugar. But these diets made me *miserable!* And were they really correct? Must we really cut out all grains and refined carbohydrates in order to live long healthy lives? Both of my grandmothers lived well into their 90s. My grandmother-in-law died at the age of 100. All three of these women were keen bakers, making cakes and biscuits, pies and scones and eating these goodies almost every day of their long lives.

I just wanted to eat the foods I loved, in normal quantities, and still have a nice slim body. An impossibility it seemed, *unless I could make fasting work.*

So once again, I turned to intermittent fasting. It was the obvious answer – no harsh regimes, no stupid expensive foods to buy. Booze and cake at the weekends! – it was perfect on paper. I resolved to read and research, to add to it, alter it, tweak it and find a way to *make* intermittent fasting work. I was determined to find out what I was doing wrong (if anything). I decided that if I could only lose half a pound a fortnight, it would be enough.

And so I began to research fasting – not in any scientific way, but in a completely human-based, anecdotal way. To be honest, I didn't want to hear from more doctors. I didn't want to see double blind peer-reviewed trials, or read about experiments done on rats. I wanted to hear from *dieters*, from other 40 year old women, *ordinary people*. I wanted to speak, both to those who were having a lot of success with intermittent fasting, and to those who were having trouble. In particular, I wanted to speak to those who had come through those same initial difficulties, and found a way to *make it work*.

I read every book on fasting, but I also spent long hours on online forums, chatting and learning from people just like me – people with genuine stories, genuine solutions and genuine results.

I discovered that I wasn't alone in my fast diet difficulties. There were thousands of people, just like me, apparently doing everything right, but not having any success with weight loss.

I learned all sorts of tips and tricks for making fasting easier and more successful. Some of these ideas I discovered for myself, from my own experience. But many are ideas I have picked up from others – things that would never have occurred to me.

I was surprised to learn that I was actually making small but crucial mistakes with my fasting.

I discovered that by changing something as simple as the time at which I ate my 500 calories made an enormous difference to my weight loss.

I discovered ways to make the hunger much easier to cope with and the best ways of keeping going when things got tough.

But best of all, I discovered all the variations. I discovered that 5:2 was not the only form of intermittent fasting. There were 4:3, 16:8, 19:5 and Alternate Day Fasting. More than anything, it was my understanding of these variations that led to my eventual success. My understanding of these enabled me to tweak things and create a programme of my own – one which fitted *my life;* one which worked *for me.* One which allowed me to continue to enjoy being the greedy, food-lover I was – just not all the time.

Before we go on, be warned: I am going to give you very few words about the health benefits or the science behind fasting. I am not a doctor or a medical professional so any knowledge I do have in this area is somewhat second-hand. If you want to read the scientific evidence for the incredible benefits to health and longevity of intermittent fasting, please see the section on suggested reading at the back of this book.

These are just two of the many perfectly good books written about each of those variations of intermittent fasting.

So why another one?

This book is written as a *helper*; it is a companion book. It is written to discuss the pros and cons, not just of **one** of these plans, not just 5:2 *or* 16:8 *or* Alternate Day Fasting, but of all of them, side by side and in conjunction with each other. It is written to help you through the psychological side of fasting – to help you through the hunger, the boredom, the weaker moments, the side-effects. It is written as a guidebook to enable you to create *your own programme* for weight loss, all based on variations of intermittent fasting.

If you are one of the very many people who doesn't seem to lose weight doing normal 5:2, this book will suggest various ways in which you may have been going wrong. And for those of you who have been doing everything right and *still* had little success with intermittent fasting, it will show you ways of combining, tweaking, and tricks and tips for making your fasting easy and your weight loss as fast and permanent as possible.

So if you have tried 5:2 fasting but didn't lose any weight, *read on.*

If you have tried some form of fasting but really struggled with the hunger, *read on.*

If you know that diets aren't the answer, and know that you need to change the way you eat, but can't resist the foods you love, *read on.*

Without gaining the knowledge I am sharing with you today, I would never have had the wonderful success, the wonderful weight loss and the trim fit body that intermittent fasting has now given me. So don't worry if you have been unsuccessful so far. It is for people like you that I wrote this book. I want you to *make it work* and if I can do it, so can you.

5:2 is only the beginning…

2 WHY FAST?

Intermittent fasting is one of the easiest, most healthy and cheapest ways to lose weight currently available. Here are just some of the benefits of this wonderful way of eating:

1. It's actually *good for you* (and may even increase your overall life expectancy).

2. It's far cheaper than any other healthy diet. While following an intermittent fasting programme you are free to eat the same food you normally would, just less of it. So you will not be required to buy special foods or expensive items. After a few weeks of this way of eating, you will see the difference it makes to your grocery bill.

3. You can eat cakes, chocolate, alcohol, crisps and still lose weight. (Although you may well find you will have far less interest in these things, once you have been fasting for some time).

Be aware: I am not suggesting you live on junk and chocolate. I am suggesting that while intermittent fasting, it is possible to eat treats on your non-fasting days and still lose weight. It is possible to be *very* greedy (as I definitely am) and still have a slim, fit body.

Now, there are all sorts of arguments for *not* eating these apparently unhealthy foods. But I am not here to discuss the health implications of eating cake or crisps – there are other books that do that job.

This book is about *weight loss.*

I'm not going to tell you what you should and shouldn't eat because I am not an expert in nutrition (if such a person exists). I *think* I eat well. And I think you should eat well, too. But I don't tend to believe the current 'healthy' food advice dogma very strongly – it changes far too often to be taken seriously. So I don't think anyone has the right to lecture us over our eating, especially when the advice given today contradicts the advice given a year ago. I take a more pragmatic approach to healthy eating. If it feels right and good for me, then I eat it. And by that reckoning, anything that makes you *feel* as good as intermittent fasting does *must* be good for you.

The way I see it is this: if someone is going to eat those junky types of food anyway, they might as well do something like fasting two days a week and receive all the weight loss and health benefits this affords.

4. You can still have an active social life with dinner parties, picnics and lunches with friends, without having to pick the boring items from the buffet, and without avoiding dessert.

5. You don't have to fight cravings all the time. *You just have to fight them for one day.* In most cases, no matter how hungry you are, or how much you are craving a particular food, *you only have to get through one day before you can have it.*

6. Intermittent fasting doesn't get boring. Most diets become dull and it becomes increasingly difficult to find the motivation to continue with them. Motivation is easy while intermittent fasting. There is always the reward of the next day to look forward to.

7. The weight you do lose will never just be water weight. With most strict diets you tend to see an initial big weight loss usually attributed to losing mere 'water weight'. When you start a crash diet you quickly empty your digestive system of carbohydrates. Carbohydrates absorb and hold a lot of water. Fewer carbohydrates in the body equals less water in the body. This explains that initial 'water weight' lost in the first few days of a diet.

With intermittent fasting the majority of your week is spent eating normally, carbs included. This means there is never a large carbohydrate loss in your body. Weight loss is real, it is fat; you are genuinely getting lighter, thinner, healthier.

8. Intermittent fasting is an *achievable* lifestyle change. We are constantly told that 'diets don't work' and the only way to consistent and permanent weight loss is to have a whole new way of eating; in other words, a 'lifestyle change'. Personally speaking, these lifestyle changes have never appealed to me. Giving up all sugar, cutting out all simple carbs, raw food, no wheat or dairy, even portion control is not something I want to be doing every day. I'm just too greedy, and too much of a food-lover for that.

Don't get me wrong: most of the time I eat very well. I cook from scratch and eat loads of vegetables. I don't have a massively sweet tooth, but I like an occasional dessert. I avoid processed food and fast junky food. I want to eat healthy food, but I want to eat *lots* of it! I want to be able to eat a blow-out roast dinner on Sundays and a cake with my Costa coffee, just because I fancy it. With intermittent fasting, that's exactly what you can do. You just can't do it every day. This is why, for most people, intermittent fasting is not a diet in the usual sense. If you are anything like me, you will find this is the one manageable, doable, enjoyable lifestyle change you are able to make.

3 BUSTING THE MYTHS ABOUT FASTING

When you tell people you have started intermittent fasting, you will often get less-than-positive responses. People will tell you that that fasting causes your metabolism to shut down and go into a sort of hibernation mode, that fasting is dangerous, that it is just another health fad like all the others out there. Let's bust a few of those myths.

Myth No. 1 – It's just another health fad.
'Why not just eat healthily and exercise?' say the doubters. If you are one of those many, many people who have always eaten healthily, have

always exercised, and have always had a weight problem, you have my sympathies. I am the same. I cook fresh food every night – not takeaways. I eat maybe one bar of chocolate a year. I exercise all the time. I used to run 7km every day until my knees gave out. And I have watched my weight creep up and up. No matter how self-righteously the doubters state 'just eat healthily and exercise' I can promise you, it doesn't *always work.*

The simple truth is, intermittent fasting does *work!* And unlike other forms of dieting, intermittent fasting is something that we can often manage to stick to for months and months without falling off the wagon in any major way. This is not a quick fix diet. It really is a way of life.

Myth No.2 – Fasting is bad for you.
Oh, *please!* I won't go deeply into the health benefits of fasting because I'm not a doctor and there are other books that do that job much better than I ever could. Suffice to say: fasting has the following incredible health benefits according the literature I have read:

- Fasting helps to normalise your insulin sensitivity. Insulin *resistance* occurs when your insulin sensitivity becomes low. This resistance contributes to nearly all chronic disease; not just diabetes but also heart disease and even cancer.

- Fasting helps to reduce inflammation in the body.

- Fasting lessens damage from free radicals which are a big contributor to all forms of cancer.

- Fasting promotes production of the human growth hormone (HGH). Sometimes called 'the fitness hormone' or the 'aging hormone', HGH plays an important part in health and fitness by speeding up the metabolism, burning fat and increasing muscle growth. As if that weren't enough, this wonderful hormone actually **slows the aging process**.

- The weight loss that occurs through fasting a couple of days a week is not achieved simply through the calorie deficit this creates. The weight loss while fasting is caused by stronger insulin sensitivity, increased HGH secretion *plus* a calorie deficit. It is all *three* of these factors combined which makes intermittent fasting so healthy and effective for long term weight loss.

But don't judge this way of eating on what a bunch of scientific studies say. *Try it and feel the benefits.* Notice the increase in energy, the improved concentration, the clearer skin, the lack of intestinal bloating and the loss of interest in sweet things. See how *good* you feel while intermittent fasting and then decide whether fasting is bad for you.

Even though fasting has been part of many cultures for millennia, the incredible health benefits of this way of eating are only just beginning to be understood by western medicine.

Think about it. Our modern way of living is very new in terms of human history. Our modern way of *eating* is even newer. Do you think our Palaeolithic ancestors had access to food 24/7? Do you think they had big breakfasts, three meals a day, afternoon snacks plus midnight fridge-raiding? Intermittent fasting is probably far closer to a 'natural' way of eating – the way of eating for which we have evolved. Perhaps one day we will evolve to be able to eat junk, tons of sugar and stuff our faces all day, *and not lose weight*. But we aren't there yet. And until we are there, you and I are going to have to do something else if we want to stay slim.

Despite all the reported health benefits, despite how good it makes you feel, and despite your shrinking waistline, sooner or later, someone will probably ask you the following:

Are you sure it's safe?

It's so funny – I used to write Facebook statuses saying things like

Just ate a whole bucket of KFC!

Blimey, turns out three bottles of red wine was too much for me after all!

Family size pack of Mars Bars? I take that as a challenge!

And when I wrote these posts, I would inevitably get comments of the following sort:

Haha! Well done. Go girl! Sounds like a good weekend!

But if I write down I am trying a juice fast (something else I like to do from time to time when I have the willpower), or that I am starting on a regime of intermittent fasting, I will get these types of responses:

Are you sure that's safe, you had better check with a doctor, why not just eat healthily and exercise?

Incredible!

Let the doubters doubt. Ignore them. Or wait until you have lost a stone to tell them you are fasting. They then won't find it so easy to criticise.

Myth No.3 – Fasting puts you in hibernation or starvation mode and you stop losing weight. The idea that normal low calorie dieters rapidly enter a starvation mode where their metabolism slows down, their bodies begin to 'shut down' and they burn fewer calories is something of a myth. Few of us will ever have entered this starvation mode, even while on very low calorie diets. It is true that those who have suffered severe calorie restriction for long periods of time have eventually adapted to using slightly fewer calories and becoming a little slower in terms of metabolism. But those findings actually came from studies of those who had spent around three *months* on severely reduced calories.

Because you are only ever fasting for a day (two at most) before eating normally again, there is simply no time for your body to enter starvation mode. In fact, when it comes to short-term fasting (up to 3 days), studies show that the metabolic rate of the participants actually tends to *increase.*

Myth No.4 – Breakfast is the most important meal of the day/breakfast kick starts your metabolism. Some of the variations in this book will involve your skipping breakfast and eating later in the day.

But isn't this terribly bad for you?

'Breakfast like a king' so the saying goes. 'Breakfast will kick start your metabolism and burn off an extra 100 calories' is another. This is such an established dogma that it might be the hardest myth of all to bust.

Looking at my own experience, I skipped breakfast for all of the early part of my life. I just never fancied food early in the morning. When I was a child, a teenager and a young woman, I never ate breakfast. No matter how many people told me it was the most important meal of the day, I wouldn't listen. I just couldn't stomach eating early in the morning. Until I was around 24 I weighed around 8 stone. When I met my husband, he was a big breakfast eater. And so, I began to eat breakfast too. It became a habit. And at age 40, I tipped the scales at 11st 6lbs. It may be coincidence but I started to put on a lot of weight at the same time that I began to eat regular breakfasts. Is it possible that that simple action of adding breakfast to my day over 15 long years, has created my entire weight loss problem? It took considerable effort to get out of the habit of eating breakfast, but now I am back to not being able to stomach food any time before about 11.

The truth is, even a moderate breakfast will always contain more calories than the supposed calorie deficit that the boost in metabolism will give. By eating breakfast you will almost always consume more calories overall – simple as that.

Additionally, most people find that eating breakfast on a fast day increases hunger later and thus makes the day more difficult to get through, not better. And as for the supposed health benefits of a big breakfast, they may be nothing more than propaganda put about by cereal manufacturers. I'm not going to blind you with science but suffice to say, plenty of recent research suggests that skipping breakfast is far better for health and weight loss than the previous dogma of eating a big breakfast. If you would like to research this for yourself, I can recommend visiting www.mercola.com.

But I still say: go with what suits *you*. Some people really feel they need a hearty breakfast and can't really function well without it (my mother is one of them). If you can't do without breakfast, that's fine. There will still be a variation of intermittent fasting that will suit you. Feel free to continue to eat in the morning, but don't discount the idea of skipping breakfast based solely on supposed health or weight loss arguments.

4 THE EATING PLANS

For those of you who may not have of intermittent fasting at all, I will very quickly run through the various types of intermittent fasting and offer guidance for following each of them.

Intermittent fasting is simply a way of eating whereby sets limits on the times at which one eats.

Sometimes this is an hourly restriction every day – whereby you consume all your calories within a certain timeframe – an eating window, every day. We will cover those eating plans a little later in the book.

The more popular form of intermittent fasting involves either fasting completely, or eating a very small amount for one, two or three days per week, but then eating normally for all the other days in between.

5:2 FASTING

The most popular form of intermittent fasting is the famous 5:2 fast diet. It is incredibly simple. For two days per week you either fast completely (ie, eat nothing at all) or, more usually, you eat a very small number of calories. For the remainder of the week, 5 days, you eat normally.

The one part of this plan which must be adhered to strictly is the calorie allowance. The fasting calorie allowance is normally a *maximum* of 500 calories for a woman and 600 for a man. These amounts are based on a calculation of one quarter the amount of a normal day's calorie requirement (2000 for a woman and 2400 for a man).

Of course, we are all different shapes and sizes. But these amounts seem to work for the majority of people.

FAST DAYS: Eat 500 calories per day, 600 if you are a man
ALL OTHER DAYS: Eat normally

Some people prefer to eat nothing on their fast days. This is absolutely fine and research shows that it is completely healthy. But for most people, going without food for an entire day and night is too difficult to sustain long term.

Many people get hung up over whether it is best to run the two days concurrently or to separate them. The answer is to choose which is easiest for you. There seems to be some evidence to suggest that those who separate the days lose a tiny bit more weight than those who fast for two consecutive days. But if fasting consecutively allows you to stick to this way of eating, do it. This is a way of life, and whatever allows you to stick to the plan long term is right for you. For a fuller explanation of this ground-breaking eating plan, see *The Fast Diet* by Dr Michael Mosley and Mimi Spencer.

4:3 FASTING

As you have probably guessed, 4:3 fasting is exactly the same as 5:2 fasting except that you fast for three days per week rather than only two. Most people who follow this programme will fast Monday, Wednesday, Friday and then can enjoy a 'normal' weekend but this is entirely personal.

FAST DAYS: Eat 500 calories per day, 600 if you are a man

ALL OTHER DAYS: Eat normally

4:3 is often popular with those who want a quick burst of weight loss at the beginning of a new regime. The weight loss will be faster than with 5:2. But bear in mind that if you are just starting out, and have never fasted before, 4:3 may not be the best way to start. You will be in danger of giving up and breaking your fast by eating. Far better is to ease yourself into fasting slowly, get used to the feeling of hunger and to discover the tricks that work best for you.

ALTERNATE DAY FASTING or ADF

Alternate Day Fasting has been written about extensively in the excellent book, *The Every Other Day Diet* by Dr Krista Varady.

The idea here is to fast *every other day*. This results in a rapid, but healthy and sustainable weight loss. Some of the original studies on longevity were done using Alternate Day Fasting and the results suggest it is an extremely healthy way to eat.

EVERY OTHER DAY: Eat 500 calories per day, 600 if you are a man
ALL OTHER DAYS: Eat normally

The drawbacks of Alternate Day Fasting are that it is much more difficult to stick to – you only ever get one day of normal eating before having to fast again – and this makes it far more difficult to fit into normal life. The programme follows a fortnightly repeating pattern, rather than weekly. This means that one week you will be fasting on Monday, Wednesday, Friday, Sunday, and the following week you will be eating on all those days. This can make it difficult to fit into the normal weekly routine.

The joy of 5:2 and 4:3 is that birthdays, parties, weddings, picnics, anniversaries and enjoyable social occasions can all be easily accommodated. When on most slimming diets, these occasions involve either not eating anything, avoiding all the most delicious foods, or eating just a tiny bit. With 4:3 and 5:2, it is always possible to shift your days one week to allow for normal eating on these social occasions. For example, if you have a birthday dinner to attend on Friday but Friday is your normal fasting day, you can just shift fasting to Saturday and no harm is done. You can go to your party, eat what you like, safe in the knowledge that tomorrow is a fast day. *And you will still lose weight!*

With Alternate Day Fasting, there is not this flexibility. Shifting days would involve your having to fast two days running, and on Alternate Day Fasting, this would be super-tough.

For most people, Alternate Day Fasting is nothing more than a quick-fix, to be followed for a few weeks or a month at most, before reverting back to a less harsh regime after a nice chunk of weight loss. But if you have the discipline to stick to this for longer, you could see a very nice weight loss indeed.

5 WHEN IT DOESN'T WORK

For many people, following simple 5:2 or 4:3 is enough. All they need do is limit their calorie intake to 500/600 calories per day, twice a week. No other restriction or rule is needed to see an acceptable weight loss.

But for some, things aren't that simple. For some, the weight does not drop off. In fact, some even manage to put weight *on* while following one of these plans. How can this possibly happen?

Below are some of the common ways in which we sometimes inadvertently scupper our chances of success with intermittent fasting.

1. Cheating on calories. I know that few of you will consciously be cheating. But inadvertent overeating does need to be mentioned before we go on. With a diet such as Weight Watchers or Slimming World, the odd apple or banana here and there, the sugar in tea three times a day, the crispbread when you are extra hungry, the stock cube in a dull soup, or nibbling at the kids' leftovers, are not such a problem. With intermittent fasting, these things can mean the difference between good weight loss and none at all.

Take the following example, if you are an average woman, and are trying to stick to 500 calories on fast days, a banana and two sugars in your tea could put your calories up by a staggering 150. That is 25% over your daily allowance.

The answer is to get used to counting *everything*. Measure your splash of milk and work out its calories. Include every single thing you eat in your total.

Get an electronic scales and weight every single thing you intend to put in your mouth. 'Manual' scales are often nowhere near accurate enough. I now weigh everything, including spices, leafy vegetables and stock. Yes, it is a bit of an inconvenience to be weighing, but it's nothing compared to the benefits of this way of eating. If you just can't face weighing your food, eat pre-packaged meals *only.* As the calories will be written on the side of the box, there will be no possibility of making a mistake.

2. Not moving at all. It is not essential to be doing huge amounts of exercise while fasting. But don't make the mistake of doing the complete opposite and barely moving all day. If your activities levels drop substantially on fast days, you will have a harder time losing the weight. Keep moving, keep active and keep your metabolism up. See also the later section on exercise.

3. Stuffing your face the night before. Some people stick religiously to their 500 calorie allowance on fast days. But the night before, they bulk up right until bedtime on food to ensure they don't feel hungry in the morning. To make matters worse, the day after the fast, these same people often have an enormous breakfast at 7am, whether they are hungry or not. If these two meals at either end of the fast are really high in calories, they will cancel out almost all the calorie restriction of the fast days. There will also be little chance of your normalising insulin levels and increasing HGH levels. Thus all these other weight loss benefits will be lost and you will be left with just a very small calorie deficit. This is unlikely to be enough to give you a satisfactorily fast weight loss.

And far from preventing morning hunger, oddly things often work in reverse. Most of us have experienced that strange phenomenon of being extra hungry the morning after a huge meal. And you'll soon find that the morning after a fast day you are often far less hungry than normal, sometimes disappointingly so!

4. Going crazy on your 'eating days' Are you making up for all the hardship of the day before by bingeing? Do you call your normal eating days 'feast days'? Don't use the lack of restriction as an excuse to eat more junk and bigger portions than you normally would. Just listen to your body, eat when hungry. If you fancy something 'naughty' like crisps or cake, then eat it. But you don't have to eat the whole family-sized bag of crisps, nor the whole cake. Do your best to eat 'normally' on your eating days. You may well find that you naturally start to eat less, crave sugar less and choose healthier food. This is a common occurrence amongst long-term intermittent fasters.

Some people have found they are more successful if they stick to a calorie limit on their eating days too. Often, this is based not on an arbitrary calorie total, but on a calculation of Total Daily Energy Expenditure or TDEE. TDEE is the number of calories required to fuel your body through its normal daily activities without losing weight. This will obviously vary from person to person and will depend on your current weight and height and your activity level. You can find resources online for calculating your TDEE. One helpful site is www.fastdiet.co.uk.

The idea is to calculate your own personal Total Daily Energy Expenditure, and to eat no more than this amount on your normal eating days. TDEE is often far *less* than the usual 2000 calories for women and 2400 for men. On fasting days you should have just a quarter of this amount instead of the usual arbitrary 500/600 calories.

But many people (me included) find this way of eating completely unacceptable. What is the point of all the hardship of a fast day if I have to keep to a calorie limit on normal days too? If I have to pay attention to my calories on eating days too, weighing and measuring everything I eat, and restricting what I eat *every day*, it is all starting to sound suspiciously like a normal calorie-controlled weight-loss diet. And we all know how unsustainable those diets are.

The good news is, there is an easier and usually far more effective way to make intermittent fasting work.

5. Not fasting for long enough. When things aren't working for you, despite keeping active and absolutely no cheating on the calories allowance, nor overeating on your days off, the place to look is in the number of hours you spend in complete fasting. By 'complete fasting', I mean those hours where you eat *nothing at all,* not 500 calories, not a tiny breakfast, but *nothing.*

The primary, but probably totally unexpected reason for not losing weight while intermittent fasting, is not going completely without food for long enough. We cover this idea in detail in the next chapter.

6 HOW TO ACCELERATE YOUR WEIGHT LOSS – EATING WINDOWS and 24 HOUR FASTS

Like many of you, I found that simple 5:2 alone didn't work very well. Weight loss was painfully slow or non-existent. But things all changed when I began to experiment with the *timings* of my eating, not just on fast days but on non-fast days, too.

Enter the 'eating window' eating plans.

What is an 'eating window'? This simply refers to the hours in the day that you are allowed to eat. Having a set eating window means *all* calories must be consumed within a set timeframe. Sticking to a shorter eating window means that the time spent eating nothing at all is far, far greater. There are several variations.

16:8

These numbers 16 and 8 simply refer to the number of hours you should spend completely fasting (16 hours), compared those you are allowed to eat (8 hours). Note that with these daily eating window plans, the *first* digit in the ratio '16:8' refers to the number of hours that you fast, not the number of hours you eat.

So, while following 16:8, you consume no calories *at all* for 16 hours out of every 24. All food and drink (except water, tea, coffee and diet drinks) must be consumed within an 8 hour time period. This could be any consecutive 8 hours during the day. For most people 11am-7pm or 12 noon-8pm work best. Simply skipping breakfast and avoiding after-dinner snacks is usually all that is required.

ALL DAYS: Eating is not restricted by calories but you must eat all of your day's food within one 8-hour time period.

However, it is important to note that you should not see the eight hour window as a complete free-for-all in terms of eating. If you eat an enormous fast food lunch, followed by snacking all afternoon and a similarly huge evening meal, skipping breakfast is going to have a minimal effect on your weight loss. So eat what you like, but be sensible.

Some people find that doing 16:8, 7 days a week, will allow them to lose weight without other restriction and without any true 'fasting' days. But most people will have to combine with 5:2 or 4:3. Of all the things that sped up my eventual weight loss, changing my 'eating window' and combining 5:2 with 16:8 had the greatest effect.

19:5 OR 'FAST FIVE'

As the name suggests, this simply means restricting further, eating in only a 5 hour window and eating nothing at all for 19 hours out of every 24. This is a good idea for those who find skipping breakfast easy and most people will lose weight by following this plan alone. But for many, it is just too restrictive.

24 HOUR FASTS REQUIRED

More recent scientific research suggests that for maximum weight loss and health benefits, a *complete* fast of a full 24 hours is needed. There should be no calorie intake during this 24 hour period. Remember it's not just the calorie restriction which causes the weight loss. We are also looking to normalise insulin levels and increase production of HGH. Without a full 24 hour fast, many people will not be successful in achieving these other fat-burning benefits.

This is not as difficult as it sounds. The way to do this is effectively to start counting the hours on the evening *before* a fast. For example, if you eat at 7pm the night before a fast, you then don't eat anything until your normal dinner at 7pm the next day. This means that if you wake up at 7am, you are already half way through! You now just have to find a way to hold off eating until dinner time at 7pm.

To ease gently into this way of eating you could simply try adding in a couple of 24 hour fasts to your week without any further counting or calorie restriction. Just eat your normal-sized meals. Two 24 hour fasts per week is enough for many people to achieve great weight loss without having to pay any attention to calorie counts. One book which describes this way of eating is *Eat Stop Eat* by Brad Pilon. See www.eatstopeat.com

24 HOUR FASTS PLUS 5:2

The next step on from simple 24 hour fasts is also to add in the restriction of eating only 500 calories on those fast days. This in effect, gives you a full 24 hour fast, broken with a small meal of 500/600 calories. This means that if you eat at 7pm on the night before a fast, you should not eat until 7pm the following night, just like with a normal 24 hour fast. But this time, when the fast is over, you eat only 500/600 calories.

Sound horrible? It's not really. As I mentioned earlier, if you wake at 7am, you are already half way through your fast. And 500/600 calories really makes a very decent sized plate of food which should see you easily through the night until morning.

Personally, I found this was the very first step towards a really successful weight loss. On fast days, I still have nothing but coffee, tea and water throughout the day and just one evening meal of 500 calories around 7.30pm.

7 YOUR FIRST FAST

I realise that many of those reading this book will already be very familiar with fasting, and may decide to skip this chapter. But I hope you don't; even those who are very experienced with fasting may still learn something from this little section.

If you have never fasted before, I recommend you plan just one fast day. If you can manage to add in a second fast during the week, then do so. But what isn't a good idea is to plough straight into doing Alternate Day Fasting or even 4:3. As I've said elsewhere, the chances of failure are too great if you do too much too soon. It is far better to give your body and mind a chance to get used to the feeling of fasting before going for the more difficult options.

It is not a good idea to be shopping and making meal plans on the day of a fast when your hunger is likely to get the better of your good judgement. Have your meal plans worked out in advance.

Breakfast, or skip it? For your very first fast, just go with your gut feeling on this (pardon the pun). If you are someone who is used to skipping breakfast, or who just doesn't tend to feel very hungry in the mornings, then I highly recommend you attempt the full 24 hour fast, and try to hold off eating until dinner time in the evening. If you become ravenously hungry by lunchtime, then have a small lunch of perhaps 150-200 calories at this time. This will still leave 300/400 calories for your evening meal.

However, if you are someone who really enjoys breakfast and feel you couldn't possibly go without in the morning, then eat a small breakfast of around 150-200 calories. A protein breakfast involving eggs and vegetables is likely to keep you feeling satisfied for longer. A mushroom or tomato omelette is ideal.

The most important thing about your first few fasts is a simple one

– don't eat something just because you feel hungry!

It's amazing how many people fail at fasting simply because they are so unused to the feeling of hunger and feel compelled to eat as soon as hunger kicks in. Because we are so unfamiliar with the feeling of real hunger, for many of us it signals danger and a desperate need to eat, *now!* Given time, the feeling of hunger loses all these negative connotations. Sure, being very hungry isn't pleasant and we all still feel the desire to eat when we are very hungry. But the desperate, ravenous, almost panicky need to eat will soon disappear. You'll be left with just perfectly normal hunger, and only ever for a few hours.

The transition from eating whenever and wherever you like, to intermittent fasting can be a bit of a shock to the system. Some people become low in energy, unable to concentrate, ravenously hungry and have side-effects such as headaches. But once through the transition, your body will adapt and you will very quickly become used to eating in this different way. You may even begin to feel sharper and more energetic on your fast days (a common effect of intermittent fasting).

My first few fasts resulted in insomnia, constipation and a low mood. But these unwanted side-effects are now just a distant memory. I now actually sleep *better* on the night after a fast, perhaps because my tummy isn't overly full of food.

Previously, I often had digestive discomfort – bloating, gassiness, pain and just a generally uncomfortable tum. I think perhaps I was just overworking my system – giving it food constantly, piling in more and more for it to work on before it had even had a chance to begin digesting the last lot! And thus it was complaining constantly. Now, all of these symptoms have all but disappeared and I am happy to report that my digestive system really seems to like this way of eating. It is only if I eat junk and lots of it, that I get a problem with my tummy these days.

Remember, these first few fasts and perhaps even the first couple of weeks of fasting are really all about getting used to the feeling of being hungry; working out the best time to eat, finding out the best things to eat, and finding out what the ideal distractions are *for you*. So don't feel too down if these first couple of weeks' worth of fasting are very difficult, or even if you feel compelled to cheat once or twice. You will settle into things and everything will very soon become easier.

8 TRICKS AND TIPS
HOW TO HAVE AN EASY AND SUCCESSFUL FAST

(read this if tempted to cheat)

1. Plan, plan, plan. If you have never fasted before, the most important thing you must do is *plan*. Plan exactly what you are going to eat and when. Get the food in beforehand. Don't leave it until the day of the fast to decide what you are going to eat because you will make bad choices. Don't ever attempt to shop for food on a fast day. I can do that now, but in the beginning passing the bread and cake shelf was torture.

Plan the meals you will eat. If cooking from scratch, plan your recipes. For great ideas, see *Fast Cook: Delicious low-calorie recipes to get you through your Fast Days* by Mimi Spencer.

2. Build up slowly. I recommend you attempt to get into the habit of eating just once a day on fast days. But this may be too difficult at first. Just go with what feels most intuitively correct for your first fast. If you feel that waiting to eat until 7pm will be best for you (perhaps because you can't do without your nice dinner) then try that. If you know you will have trouble missing breakfast, have a small meal in the morning and save the rest for later. These first few fasts will be all about getting used to things – getting used to hunger, getting used to not eating automatically, getting used to weighing and measuring.

3. Forget the weekly weigh.
If you have ever attended Weight Watchers, Slimming World or followed any type of diet plan you will no doubt have been told that daily

weighing is a big no-no. Because weight can fluctuate from hour to hour and day to day, weekly weighing is preferable because it gives a more accurate picture of your genuine weight loss.

Can you see the contradiction here?

If your weight can vary by as much as 4lbs day to day, then this is also true of weekly weighing. Let's say you have been following intermittent fasting for one whole week. You jump on the scales on a Monday and it shows a weight gain of 2lbs from the previous Monday. This is a real blow to your confidence and you feel crestfallen; after all, you have been so good. How could you have put 2lb *on?* But think about it: you could just be at the far end of one of those big fluctuations. If you had weighed the previous day, you could have shown a *loss* of 2lbs instead!

As we are only looking at overall weight losses of around 1-2lbs per week, these fluctuations could make weekly weighing highly inaccurate for a whole month!

The most accurate way to measure your weight loss success is daily, but charting a trend, rather than measuring actual success day to day. It can help to create a weight loss graph chart and to plot a line of your weight loss. This will show the general trend downwards, even when daily fluctuations may be large.

Personally, I like to weigh, not every day, but every day *after a fast*. Because I tend to eat almost exactly the same thing on fast days, the morning after a fast my stomach is in a fairly similar state as the last weighing. There can be huge fluctuations in daily weights which have nothing to do with fat. Hormones, water and food in the stomach can all give wildly inaccurate weight readings. You can overcome some of this by only weighing the morning after a fast. This will ensure that you stomach in at a similarly empty state to the last time you weighed.

And bear in mind that weight loss can often plateau for several weeks before really kicking in again. As long as the general trend is down, be happy with your progress.

As I am now down to my perfect weight, I rarely weigh any more. I fast only one day per week as a maintenance measure, only occasionally going back up to two days after having a particularly greedy weekend, or a holiday. Sometimes, I even eat breakfast, if I really fancy it. But with only one day's fasting and doing 16:8 only most of the time, it's amazing how level my weight is these days. Whenever I jump on the scales, I seem to be exactly the same weight. What a 'diet' this is!

It can also help to take measurements rather than going only on the word of the scales. Many people find they lose inches before they see a change on the scales. Don't bother with arms and legs and all sorts of complicated readings. Just measure the distance around your tummy, using your belly button as a permanent marker of where the measuring tape should go. I know this is not officially your 'waist' but it is a fixed point on your body. If the measurement around your belly button is decreasing, you are succeeding.

4. Drink Water. Drink *lots* of water! The obvious benefit of this is that water fills your stomach, giving the sensation of fullness and helping stave off hunger pangs. What you may not realise is that dehydration can also cause you to feel more hungry than normal. Sometimes, when we feel hungry, our bodies are actually craving water, not food. So drinking lots of water will have a far greater effect on your hunger than you might expect.

Some of the more unpleasant side effects of fasting can be headaches and occasional constipation. These are usually just the side-effects of dehydration. Drinking plenty of water will go a long way to ensuring these unpleasant symptoms don't disrupt your fasting. You can also drink black or herbal teas, or diet drinks.

(I don't ever eat or drink products containing artificial sweeteners because I am worried about possible effects on health. There are many arguments against consuming diet drinks and that aspartame in particular may be very bad for you.

See www.mercola.com for details. I leave you to do the research and make up your own mind.)

If you really cannot stomach any more water or tea, try a spoonful of Bovril or a stock cube dissolved in water (around 10-15 calories). It makes a tasty salty snack which can be very effective in staving off hunger and getting rid of any headache. Later in the book I also have a list of very low calorie foods which you can use to keep the hunger pangs at bay.

5. Eat only one meal on fast days. As I explained earlier, eating one meal can be more effective in terms of weight loss that spreading the calories throughout the day. Michael Mosley distributed his calories throughout the day, having a small breakfast, skipping lunch and having a small evening meal. But you may find that fasting completely (eating nothing) all day, and then having one decent-sized meal at a normal dinner time not only works better for slimming, but that it actually makes hunger easier to deal with. Given time to get used to the restriction, most people find eating once becomes *easier* than spreading the calories throughout the day. Don't believe it? Neither did I at first. The thought of missing breakfast, lunch and not eating anything at all until 7pm sounded like pure torture. All I can say is *try it*. Have you ever noticed that eating breakfast makes you feel *hungrier* later in the day? Try going without. It takes a bit of getting used to, but you may soon come to see that the hunger is *easier* to deal with if you put off eating until the evening.

One unpleasant side effect is an inability to sleep the night after a fast, particularly in the early days. Eating a good sized evening meal will ensure that you do not go to bed ravenously hungry and sleep will be far easier to come by.

But the main draw for me of eating one meal on fast days is the knowledge that I can have a really good dinner in the evening. 500 calories is a really decent plateful and this keeps me motivated all day. So I get in two full 24 hour fasts during my week and I only eat 500 calories on each of those days (effectively 5:2 plus 24 hour fasts). And it really is no longer a hardship.

6. Distraction, distraction, distraction: Games, reading, gardening, housework, chatting on the phone, working on repetitive tasks, *anything* that will get your mind off your hunger – This is the key to managing fasting days. The more distracted you are, the less you will be thinking about food. Sometimes, when I am sufficiently busy and distracted, I find a fasting day can be an absolute breeze.

7. Give it time. Fasting gets far easier the more you do it. The feeling of hunger is so unfamiliar to many of us that it can feel very uncomfortable at first and 'not right'. But it's just hunger. It won't kill you; it won't even harm you. It is actually good for you. You will find that the hungry feeling doesn't get worse as the day goes on. You don't get hungrier and hungrier. You will simply get to a certain level of hunger and stay there. Hunger also comes and goes throughout the day. With enough distraction, those moments of pure ravenous hunger become fewer. Get used to feeling hungry and it just stops feeling so bad.

I have to admit, that even now, sometimes a day comes along where things are harder. Sometimes I'm just really hungry and find it more difficult than normal. But I know it's only ever a day … I can deal with a day.

Also bear in mind that side effects such as headaches, ravenous hunger and sleeping difficulties are common during your first few weeks of fasting, but most of them will eventually disappear as you get more used to fasting.

8. Play computer games. This is my own personal tip for wiling away those long hours before the evening meal of a fast day. Computer games are my guilty pleasure. The best sorts of games are the horribly addictive online games like Tetris and Candy Crush. But you could also play Playstation or Xbox games. Two hours can pass quickly and happily and hunger pangs are forgotten when you are really into your game.

But perhaps you don't think this a productive and valuable enough use of your time…

Previous to fasting, I never allowed myself the luxury of taking two hours off to do something as stupid and pointless as play video games. I would always have felt too guilty about wasting my life. But since fasting, I have discovered the joy of allocating myself a couple of hours of pointless play. Rather than being a waste of life, I now see it as essential down-time in my busy week. I actually *look forward* to fast days because it's the only time I allow myself this useless fun.

9. Brushing your teeth can often help get you past a particularly strong craving.

10. Give yourself 30 minutes to get past a craving. If ever you are really wavering, and are in real danger of eating, do the following. Decide to wait 30 minutes without eating. Then reassess the situation. At that point, try putting off for another 30 minutes, telling yourself you can eat at the end of the time if you still really want to. Usually, by the time this hour has ticked by, the craving has lessened and the danger has passed.

Be warned: at certain points, your mind may start to try and 'trick' you into eating. You will suddenly come up with all sorts of reasons why a different diet will suddenly seem preferable. 'Atkins is the answer' or 'I really think Weight Watchers will work this time'. All that is happening is that your brain is trying to find a way to make you eat, right now. *Don't fall for the trick.* If you give in and eat something, you will regret it. And I promise you, a few hours after ruining your fast, that other diet isn't going to look so inviting after all. You will just be left with a full tummy and a lot of regret.

This is the best 'diet' in the world, don't break it

9 EXERCISE

A big mistake that fasters often make is to use the hunger of fasting as a sort of excuse to do nothing, to lounge around doing nothing, barely moving. If you do far less activity on a fast day than you would normally you are making it far harder for the calorie deficit to make a dent in your weight.

There are numerous studies done on exercising *while fasting* which show that this is an extremely effective way to lose weight, gain muscle and stay healthy. Far from being a bad thing, and in direct opposition to previous dogma, exercising on an empty stomach can be preferable to a carb-rich preparation meal.

In my opinion (and my experience) *any* exercise will do. Any movement, from a ten minute walk to an hour on a squash court will help you to speed your metabolism and burn more calories.

Exercise also acts as a great mood-lifter which can help you to get through a difficult day. I also tend to find that after exercise, I just feel so virtuous that don't want to eat rubbish, or even as much food as normal!

HIIT TRAINING

If you can manage it, try adding a couple of days of HIIT training into your week. HIIT stands for High Intensity Interval Training.

The concept of High Intensity Interval Training is simple. To do HIIT, you do a short warm up, and then you do an intense but very short burst of cardio, followed by a full recovery period. HIIT is often best done on an exercise bike or a treadmill. For example, my own HIIT exercise bike workout followed the following pattern.

1. I warmed up for 5 minutes, with gentle cycling, just to get my legs moving.

2. I then increased the bike's resistance to full and went flat out pedalling as hard as I could for 30 seconds.

3. I then gently cycled for 2 minutes to catch my breath.

4. Then another 30 seconds at full throttle.

5. Then a couple minutes gentle cycling.

6. Then the final 30 seconds at full pelt, on the highest resistance.

7. Then I *rested!*

According to the experts, this workout will burn as many calories as an hours' moderate bike ride. You will find yourself utterly exhausted after just this short exercise session. You can follow exactly the same pattern on a treadmill, sprinting for short bursts, followed by periods of walking. This is far, far more effective than plodding along on a treadmill for hours at a time and in a fraction of the time.

For a fuller explanation, tips and tricks and for the science behind this exercise method, read *Fast Exercise* by Michael Mosley and Peta Bee.

Some fans of HIIT claim it is most effective when done on the day of a fast, on a completely empty stomach. But not me. I couldn't stand to do HIIT on an empty stomach. It made me feel physically terrible and I once fainted after a HIIT session while fasting. If you want to try HIIT, I recommend you do it only on your non-fasting days, particularly in the early days. You should also consult a doctor before starting any exercise regime.

But if you can't seem to make HIIT work *at all* while fasting, don't despair. There is a far, *far* easier way to add exercise to your intermittent fasting regime.

JUST WALK

If you want an easy, low-impact, non-risky way to increase your metabolism, distract yourself from hunger, get more sunshine vitamin D, improve your mood *and* burn more fat, just walk 10,000 steps a day.

For this, you will need a pedometer. A pedometer is a fun and handy way to keep a track of your day's activity. It is also extremely motivating to have a moment-by-moment account of your steps. It will give you a real sense of satisfaction and achievement to see that total roll around to 10,000. You can buy them extremely cheaply from Amazon or elsewhere. Some even have calorie counters, which provide an additional motivating factor.* Each day, make sure you get your 10,000 steps in. This total includes walking to and from work, around the house, going to the toilet, everything. If you haven't been active enough during the day, just add in a walk around the block before or after dinner. You can even just walk around the house if it is raining outside.

*Don't ever be tempted to 'eat' the extra calories you burn and so go over your 500/600 calorie limit. Your weight loss will grind to a halt. Calories burned through exercise do NOT equal calories eaten through food.

It's amazing how the presence of that little gadget in your pocket will affect your daily activities. You'll find yourself naturally taking the long way to the canteen, walking up the stairs rather than taking the lift, walking to buy a pint of milk rather than taking the car. You'll feel better, you'll get more sunshine, and your mood will even improve. And when done consistently, preferably every day, simple walking will ramp up your weight loss so that in a few months' time, you'll be that much lighter.

10 THE QUICK GUIDE TO WINNING COMBINATIONS – HOW TO TAILOR YOUR OWN EATING PROGRAMME

I firmly believe that anyone can tweak the basic fasting patterns to come up with a programme which suits them, both in terms of fitting in with one's life, and with satisfactory weight loss.

Below are some of the most popular variations.

5:2 PLUS 16:8

This is a very common combination that works well for many people. The two fasting days are as normal – you eat just 500/600 calories two days a week. On some or all of the other days you follow 16:8 (i.e., keeping all your eating to an eight hour window). It is up to you whether to do 16:8 on all five days or whether to take a day or two off (perhaps just eating completely normally at weekends). This combination is easier than it sounds, especially considering that many people feel less hungry the morning after a fast than they normally would. Very often, you may find yourself going to bed on a fast day with thoughts full of food, thinking of all the lovely things you can eat tomorrow, knowing that when you wake you can have a nice big breakfast... but then, morning comes and all that hunger and craving seems to have disappeared! Food just doesn't seem as interesting the morning after a fast. If you have had this experience then a 5:2 and 16:8 combination is likely to be ideal for you. This also works extremely well for those who generally don't have a problem with skipping breakfast or those who usually have a late breakfast.

FAST DAYS: Eat 500 calories per day, 600 if you are a man

ALL OTHER DAYS: Eat only within an 8 hour window.

16:8 can also be combined with 4:3 or Alternate Day Fasting in exactly the same way. Obviously, these combinations are slightly tougher, but will result in faster weight loss and are still very healthy.

5:2 PLUS EXERCISE

If 5:2 fasting is all the restriction you can cope with, the answer may be to simply increase your levels of activity. Many people are combining HIIT with intermittent fasting and achieving incredible results in terms of fitness, strength and massive weight loss. If you prefer something more gentle, I highly recommend taking up walking, as I discussed earlier in the book. Add in a nice long daily walk (at least 10,000 steps in total per day) and this may be all you need to ramp up the weight loss.

FAST DAYS: Eat 500 calories per day, 600 if you are a man
ALL OTHER DAYS: Eat normally
AT LEAST 3-5 TIMES A WEEK: Exercise

5:2 BUT HAVING ALL YOUR CALORIES IN ONE MEAL A DAY
(basically, a 24 hour fast)

This is only a subtle change but one which can have a profound change on the ease and efficacy of 5:2 or 4:3 fasting. A surprising majority of people eventually find it is easier to fast all day, and then to eat one reasonable sized meal at dinner time. And, for all the biological reasons mentioned earlier, it actually can give the weight loss a boost too. One of the main benefits of eating just one meal a day is that there is a decent sized meal waiting for you in the evening. Rather than having to squeeze a decent meal out of 250-300 calories, you have a full 500/600 calories with which it is easy to make a really substantial plateful. This makes the whole day's fasting that much easier, knowing there is a filling, satisfying and delicious meal at the end of the day. This can also make sleeping far easier because you are not going to bed feeling starved.

FAST DAYS: Eat 500 calories per day, 600 if you are a man. Eat all your calories in one meal which must be 24 hours after the last time you ate.
ALL OTHER DAYS: Eat normally

HOW TO CREATE YOUR OWN EATING PLAN

While intermittent fasting, people often become hung up on the answers to questions such as

'Is it best to fast two consecutive days instead of splitting them?'

'Is it better to exercise on fast days or non-fast days?'

'I had 550 calories on a fast day, have I ruined everything?'

'Can I do 15:9 at the weekends instead of 16:8?'

'Can I have a splash of milk in my morning coffee/afternoon tea?'

The answers to all these questions is the same *if it works for your then it's right for you.*

And the only way to find this out is to try it. I have a friend who fasts just one day a week and still loses half a pound every week. She thinks it works so well because this one day's fasting has caused her to lose her previous sweet tooth and so her sugar intake has been drastically reduced.

I almost *always* go without breakfast now. Both on fast and non-fast days, I never eat before 11 or noon. But my own mother, who has also lost a lot of weight with intermittent fasting wouldn't dream of going without breakfast. She feels she simply can't function without it. My sister always fasts two consecutive days, Monday and Tuesday. She likes to get the fasting out of the way early in the week so that she can enjoy the rest of it in peace. This wouldn't work for me or my husband at all. It is the thought of being able to eat normally tomorrow that keeps us fasting today!

So as you can see, even within the same family there are big differences in fasting preferences yet we all are able to make it work.

And incidentally, I cannot *stand* black coffee or black tea. I always have a splash of milk in my morning coffee and sometime in a cup of afternoon tea as well, even in the middle of a 24 hour fast. This tiny amount of calories doesn't seem to affect my ability to lose weight. Perhaps I would lose faster if I didn't have the milk, but without the milk I might just find this eating plan unbearable. If having a splash of milk in your coffee means you stick to the plan, then drink the milk, I say!

So feel free to experiment with your own combinations.

You could do…
5:2 plus 19:5
4:3 plus HIIT training
4:3 plus 19:5
16:8 plus Alternate Day Fasting
And so on…

Generally speaking the bigger the first digit in the ratio, the faster the weight loss, for example
4:3 is faster than 5:2
5:2 is faster than 6:1
19:5 is faster than 16:8
18:6 is faster than 16:8 (this is simply a pattern where all the eating is kept to a six hour window).

Probably the ultimate hardcore regime is Alternate Day Fasting plus 19:5. Just to remind you, with 19:5, you eat just in a small five hour window. This means eating only between the hours of say, 3pm and 8pm. On fast days, you still eat only your 500/600 calories. I have done this combination now and again just for a week or two. I lose a lot of weight and I actually feel great on it. But because it is so extreme, it is really not sustainable for long periods. Life and hunger just get in the way of such a regime. It may not even be as healthy. If you fancy trying an extreme combination such as this one, always consult a doctor before doing so.

EVERY OTHER DAY: Eat 500 calories per day, 600 if you are a man
ALL OTHER DAYS: Eat normally but consume all your calories in an 8 hour window

MY OWN IDEAL

When I want to lose weight, I fast Tuesdays and Thursdays. I do 16:8 Monday, Wednesday, Thursday. On fast days I eat one meal of 500 calories at around 7.30pm (usually a huge chicken and vegetable curry with rice). This means that not only do I get two full 24 hour fasts into each week, I also only break my fast with 500 calories. This effectively means I am eating only 500 calories in a 42 hour period twice a week. *Sounds awful when you put it like that, yet it is easy!* On the other three weekdays I simply skip breakfast and eat lunch at around 12.30 and dinner at around 7 or 8. I walk 10,000 steps every single day, six or seven days a week. At the weekends I eat whatever I want, whenever I want. Not only do I find I lose weight at a nice steady speed, I find this absolutely easy and doable.

I am now at my ideal weight and only fast one day per week as a maintenance measure. But when following the above eating plan, I would lose a steady 1-2lb per week. This was exactly what I lost on Weight Watchers with much less hassle! Unlike Weight Watchers, this regime didn't interfere with my life and I never feel tempted to cheat. If a social occasion fell on a fast day, I simply shifted things around and did 16:8 on that day instead, moving my fast day to Wednesday or Friday (I never fasted two days running).

Whenever I had a hunger pang or a craving, I just told myself 'you can have it at noon,' or 'you can eat whatever you want tomorrow' and this way, I only ever needed one day's worth of willpower. In fact, although I was allowed to go wild at the weekends, I found I didn't really want to. I felt so much brighter and more energetic that I didn't always feel like ruining it all with food. Sometimes, I would really indulge, drink and eat far too much. And on those weekends, I found myself looking forward to a fast day! Fast days meant I felt less lethargic, less bloated and 'cleaner'.

The idea is not to go mad and do the harshest, hardest regime possible in order to have rapid weight loss, nor is it a good idea to do the easiest thing possible with only minimum weight loss. The idea is to find some combination that gives you a steady weight loss, but which is *sustainable!* It is sustainability that will mean you are a winner, it is this which will allow you to stick to this plan where you would normally fall off the wagon and cheat, it is sustainability that means in six months you will be a completely different size and shape, rather than two pounds heavier. Try to get your head away from *fast* weight loss and into *steady, constant* and *permanent* weight loss!

So play around with this. Start easy and build up. If you fancy a faster weight loss for a bit, go in harder. But if it turns out to be too much to cope with, don't give up on fasting. Just go back to simple 5:2 and reassess. I firmly believe that there is a way to make this work for everyone.

I recommend that everyone starts with 5:2, simply because it is one of the easiest and overall is the most successful of all the fasting plans. If you can make 5:2 work without any of the other added combinations, you are laughing. Don't get side-tracked by the idea of rapid weight loss and decide to set out to do some super hard core plan, such as 19:5 or Alternate Day Fasting. There is just too much danger that you will fail and become despondent about the whole thing. Build up slowly, finding out what works for you, what distractions work for hunger, whether one meal a day works better than 3, whether you fast better on Mondays or Tuesdays…all these things won't be known to you until you have more experience of fasting. And without knowing these things, the tougher regimes are going to be near-impossible to stick to.

11 WHAT TO EAT?

As I only eat one meal a day while fasting, I can really eat a very good sized meal in the evening. My staple dinner is a large chicken and vegetable curry with rice. My husband and I always fast together and we take it in turns to cook the curry. (His always tastes slightly different to mine!) I include the recipe below.

I'm not going to fill this book with recipes as there are far better books dedicated to that. I will just include my personal favourite. If you are like me, you will find a couple of recipes work really well for you and you will end up cooking the same couple of meals over and over.

My Delicious Chicken and Veg Curry `
(Calorie values in brackets)

200g Carrots (66)

200g Tinned chopped tomatoes (40)

100g Chopped Onions (38)

150g Cabbage (39)

100g Swede (32)

200g Supermaket-bought frozen chicken breast (check the nutritional information) or 220g Quorn Pieces (200)

2 Oxo chicken stock cubes (30)

10g Sharwoods Madras Curry Powder (32)

Spray Oil (5)

500ml water (0)

1 tsp sugar (optional but yummy) (16)

120g Basmati rice (420)

Total (serves 2)   <u>918 calories</u>

Fry off the onion in 5 sprays of oil. Chop and add all the other vegetables, the curry powder, the stock and around 500ml of water. Bring to the boil and simmer for 35 minutes. I then like to partially liquidise the curry with a hand blender to give a nice thick texture. Chop the chicken and fry off in a couple of pumps of spray oil until cooked. Then add the chicken to the curry. Cook the rice, serve and enjoy this enormous meal!

This recipe makes two 459 calorie portions (450 if you leave out the sugar). This still leaves a small allowance for a little milk in tea or coffee during the day. Men may increase the amount of chicken or rice, or add a couple of shop-bought poppadums to make up to 600 calories. My husband likes to add a banana to his curry. (Yuk!) Always remember to check the nutritional information, particularly on the chicken you are using. I tend to use the frozen bags of chicken which contain added water. These contain fewer calories than fresh chicken but seem to go further. If cooking just for yourself, either halve the ingredients or make a double portion and freeze for your next fast.

THERE ARE ALWAYS READY- MEALS

If you really can't be bothered to cook, you can't cook or you simply don't have time one day, ready meals are your friend. I did my first 3 months' fasting using Weight Watcher meals. I loved the Chicken Hotpot with a big pile of broccoli. Another great range is Marks and Spencer Fuller Longer range. The beauty of ready meals is that they inevitably have the calories listed on the packet. No need to weigh or measure. If the idea of weighing, measuring and cooking is putting you off the whole idea of intermittent fasting, just use ready meals. You can always add in some fresh vegetables for extra health benefits.

12 EMERGENCY LOW-CALORIE LIFESAVERS

An Oxo cube dissolved in water is only 16-17 calories

A tablespoonful of beef Bovril dissolved in water is only 22 calories

A tablespoonful of chicken Bovril dissolved in water is only 16 calories

Two large strawberries is only 10 calories

Ice lollies made with diet squash have zero calories

Shop-bought ice pops are usually less than 5 calories each

Some pots of sugar free jelly are only 10 calories

1 Laughing Cow Light wedge on 2 small or 1 large celery - 40 calories

A frozen Petit Filou (50g pot) is only 48 calories. You can sit and dig it with a spoon in front of the TV for a delicious, ice-creamy snack

Microwave or dry-fry 100g of beansprouts and add a tablespoon of soy sauce – only around 50 calories and utterly delicious

Rice cakes are around 35 calories

Wafer thin ham rolls with lettuce inside are around 10 calories

Large gherkins are only around 5 calories each

Certain crispbreads (Crackerbread is one) are only 19 calories (check the pack)

12 blueberries is only 10 calories

3 green or red grapes is 10 calories

18 roasted/salted sunflower seeds is 10 calories

3 plain M&Ms is 10 calories

3 cherry tomatoes is 10 calories

10 edamame (soybeans) is only 10 calories

1 large celery stick is around 10 calories

Brushing your teeth is *zero* calories but will often kill a sweet craving stone dead!

Black coffee, black tea, green tea and herbal tea contain *no* calories.

If you can't stand tea without milk, try Redbush tea (Rooibos). It tastes good without milk and has more flavour than most herbal teas.

If you are in real danger of giving up the fast and you feel a huge temptation to blow everything and eat. Try a snack AND a drink, such a Crackerbread with Marmite plus a cup of tea with a splash of milk. This is only around 40 calories but will often keep you going for many hours. This may well get you through the danger and you will be back on track.

And finally,

13 SOME MOTIVATIONAL SOUNDBITES FOR THOSE TOUGH MOMENTS

If you wake up at 7am, you'll already be halfway your 24h fast when you get up.

Your first fast is the hardest.

Fasting 2x per week for 24h cuts your calorie intake by about 30%.

Never break your fast just because you're hungry.

You can eat it tomorrow.

Don't panic about weight fluctuations, they are completely normal.

You aren't fasting, you aren't starving, you are *repairing*.

Every hour that I fast I am increasing my life expectancy.

Every hour that I fast I am getting thinner.

Your day-to-day variation in weight can be as much as 4lbs.

It's this or back to 'normal dieting' and you know how horrible that is.

Weight loss is not a smooth path, not a straight line from fat to slim. Expect jumps, dips, plateaus and wobbles.

As long as the trend is down, it's all good.

Breakfast does *not* prevent obesity.

Breakfast does *not* speed up your metabolism.

Skipping breakfast is an easy way to avoid the most high carb, high sugar meal of the day.

For many people, breakfast is *not* the most important meal of the day, it is an unnecessary meal.

Fasting for 2-3 days will *not* put you into starvation mode.

Intermittent fasting will often *increase* your metabolism.

Never beat yourself up for falling off the wagon. Just get back on the plan tomorrow and not much harm is done. This is a way of eating, a way of life, not a diet.

Side-effects such as headaches, light-headedness and trouble sleeping will lessen with time and eventually disappear.

If lack of sleep is becoming a problem, try saving some of your calories for a snack before bed. A crispbread with marmite and a caffeine-free drink can work wonders.

If you have a good book, a good film or a new computer game, save it for a fast day. Treats like this make fast days something to look forward to.

If you feel grumpy when you are hungry, this could just be the result of habit. When your body becomes familiar with the feeling of hunger, it will stop trying to make you feel grumpy.

If you are wondering whether a particular combination of fasting plans will work for you, *try it*. It's the only way to find out.

What other 'diet' allows you to eat *anything* you like, and in unlimited quantities (albeit, not *all* the time)?

This is the best 'diet' in the world.

Be good today, for tomorrow, we eat!

FURTHER READING:

The Fast Diet by Michael Mosley and Mimi Spencer

Fast Exercise by Michael Mosley and Peta Bee

Fast Cook: Delicious low-calorie recipes to get you through your Fast Days by Mimi Spencer

The 8-Hour Diet by David Zinczenko

The IF Diet by Robert Skinner

HELPFUL WEBSITES:

www.eatstopeat.com
www.mercola.com
www.fastdiet.co.uk
www.fastday.com

Made in the USA
Lexington, KY
30 May 2016